# KEGEL EXERCISES FOR WOMEN

*Beginners Guide To Kegel Exercises*
*for Vaginal Tightening, Pelvic Floor*
*Muscle Massage And Management Of*
*Female Incontinence*

**By**

# KATHERINE PALMER

# Table of Contents

# INTRODUCTION

Kegel exercises have long been used as an effective method of strengthening the pelvic floor muscles in both men and women. Unlike regular exercises that involve the full range of your muscles, kegel exercises are a bit different. Here, only one group of muscles is involved: the pelvic floor muscles.

Even more, the facts that kegels are very simple to do and can be performed anywhere, without any person's knowledge, are worth noting.

In this book, we shall try to look at how you (a woman) can perform these highly beneficial exercises in order to strengthen the kegel muscles.

I think it needs to be mentioned early on here that the key to reaping the benefits of kegel exercises is consistency. That is, repeating the exercises several times every day is necessary to get tight pelvic muscles.

# CHAPTER 1

## WHAT YOU NEED TO KNOW
## ABOUT KEGEL EXERCISES

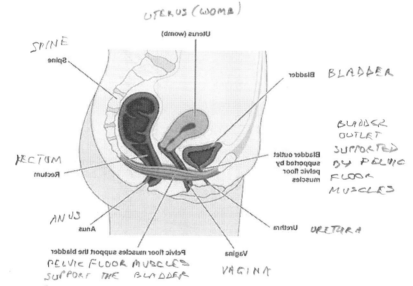

UTERUS (WOMB)

SPINE

BLADDER

BLADDER OUTLET SUPPORTED BY PELVIC FLOOR MUSCLES

RECTUM

ANUS

URETHRA

PELVIC FLOOR MUSCLES SUPPORT THE BLADDER

VAGINA

### The kegel muscles

The group of supporting structures that comprise bones, ligaments, muscles, and other connective tissues located at the pelvic region is referred to as the pelvic floor.

The pelvic floor muscles provide support for the bladder, rectum, uterus, and small intestine in women. These muscles help to hold your organs in place. Kegel exercises can help in controlling problems caused by loose or weak pelvic floor muscles – also referred to as kegel or pubococcygeus (PC) muscles.

The next section gives a brief history of kegel exercises and how you can identify the kegel muscles.

## What are Kegel Exercises?

Named after Dr. Arnold Kegel, who developed them, kegel exercises are done primarily to help in strengthening the muscles of the pelvic floor. Different factors can make the pelvic floor muscles become weak, such as childbearing, obesity, and aging.

Basically, kegel exercises involve contraction (squeezing) and relaxing of the pelvic floor muscles in succession.

These exercises can help men and women who suffer incontinence due to weak pelvic floor muscles. However, while the exercises are pretty easy, many people are not doing them correctly as they don't engage the right muscles.

## Locating the Pelvic floor muscles

Locating the pelvic muscles is the first step in practicing kegel exercises; but, the process of finding the muscles is not as easy as the exercises. The following steps will help you to achieve this.

## Method 1

Step 1: First, act as if you are trying to avoid letting out gas

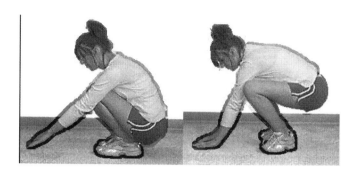

Step 2: Then, pretend to tighten your vagina around a cotton plug

You should feel the pelvic floor muscles moving up and then down after this process

## Alternative Method

Another method of locating the pelvic floor muscles is this:

i. Drink a lot of water so that it causes you to want to go ease yourself

ii. While urinating, try to stop the urine from coming out

iii. Then, allow the urine flow to resume

You can identify the kegel muscles by their contraction when stopping the urine and relaxation as you resume the flow.

After locating the kegel muscles, the subsequent steps are easier. Regardless of the reason for the exercises, the remaining steps majorly involve contracting and relaxing the kegel muscles and repeating the process.

## Techniques for Kegel Exercises

Repeating the same steps every time can be boring at times. Based on this, you can spice up your kegels using other interesting methods. The following are different ways of performing kegels for equally effective results.

# The Bridge

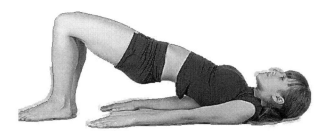

Steps

i.  Stay in the bridge position: your head and back on the floor while your hands are also on the floor. Then, start raising your hips up

ii.     Then, start to squeeze your pelvic floor muscles and relax as usual

Repeat the steps three times each week.

# The Hip Shaker

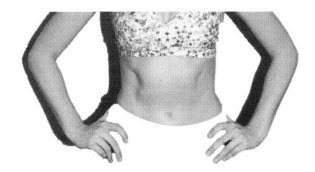

Steps

i.   Stand up with your hands on your hips and legs wide apart.

ii.  Then, start to swing your hips from one side to the other

Repeat the procedure thrice weekly for best results

## The Wall Squat

Steps

i. With your back against the wall, spread your legs apart

ii. Breathe in

iii. Then, contract your PC muscles

iv. Start to raise your pelvis up while lowering into a squat position, holding the muscles

v. Begin to stand up and relax the pelvic floor muscles when up

Rest for about ten seconds and repeat

## The Clamshell Pose

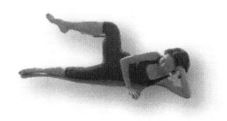

Steps

i.   Lie down on one of your sides (maybe your left side)

ii.  Next, raise your other knee up and start to move it in a circular manner

## The Endurance Test

This procedure is done to increase your endurance during kegels

Steps

  i.   Contract your pelvic floor muscles while raising your pelvis
  ii.  Stay in that position for some time

## The Quick Hit

This technique helps to improve a leaking bladder and sexual urge

Steps

i. Sit or lie down with your knees separated by a small gap

ii. Squeeze your PC muscles and relax them repeatedly in quick successions

## The Reverser

Steps

i. Contract your pelvic floor muscles as usual

ii. Then, instead of resting the muscles normally, exhale heavily when relaxing the muscles

# CHAPTER 2

## KEGEL EXERCISES FOR VAGINAL TIGHTENING

As previously stated, several factors, such as menopause, pregnancy, and aging can make a woman's vagina become loose. There are various ways that a woman can employ in tightening the muscles of her vagina. Common methods include the use of gels and surgery. Surgery may result in some unwanted side effects like nerve damage and infection. This is where kegels come into play. Kegel exercises can also be used for this purpose without complications.

## Procedure

To use kegel exercises for vaginal strengthening follow the steps below:

i. Sit with your legs crossed on a mat

ii. After locating your kegel muscles, squeeze them for about five seconds

iii. Next, allow the muscles to relax for another ten seconds. This break is necessary so that you do not strain the muscles

iv. Then, repeat the process for at least ten times for three daily sessions

*Note: Do not hold your breath while doing this. Also, note that the results*

*of the exercises may take a while to manifest, so you need to practice daily and be patient*

# CHAPTER 3: KEGEL EXERCISES FOR PELVIC FLOOR MUSCLE MASSAGE

It is possible to feel pain in the pelvic region. Kegel exercises can be used to relieve such kind of pain. The process for massaging a painful pelvic floor can be divided into two parts. The first part will help to prepare the kegel muscles for the main procedure.

## Preparing

Follow the steps below to train the pelvic floor muscles:

i. Squeeze the kegel muscles in a fast manner, stay in this position for about 2 seconds

ii. Relax the muscles for another 2 seconds

iii. Take a break and repeat steps 1 and 2 nine more times, with similar intermittent breaks

iv. Raise the pelvic floor on each consequent attempt

After you have perfected the prep exercise, you can progress to the next

**Progressing**

i. Squeeze the pelvic floor muscles as strong as you can, holding the muscles in position and further contracting

ii. Relax the muscles and start over again

iii. Repeat the process four more times, raising the pelvic floor higher on successive attempts

iv. Finally, relax the muscles to their normal position

# CHAPTER 4: KEGEL EXERCISES FOR MANAGING FEMALE INCONTINENCE

Female incontinence is a serious issue with women whose pelvic floor muscles have become loose. This problem is particularly common with women who have recently given birth.

## Types of female incontinence

Kegel exercises can be very beneficial to women who have any of the following types of incontinence:

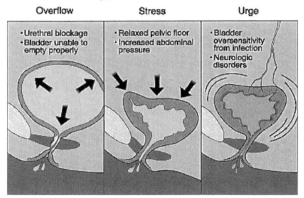

**Types of Incontinence**

| Overflow | Stress | Urge |
|---|---|---|
| • Urethral blockage<br>• Bladder unable to empty properly | • Relaxed pelvic floor<br>• Increased abdominal pressure | • Bladder oversensitivity from infection<br>• Neurologic disorders |

**Stress incontinence**, where the woman unexpectedly passes out few drops of urine while laughing, lifting, straining, or coughing.

**Fecal incontinence**: where the woman involuntarily passes out feces.

**Urge incontinence**. This is common in women older than 60 years of age. It is marked by an urgent need to urinate followed immediately by a loss of urine.

## Steps to Manage Female Incontinence Using Kegel Exercises

If you want to manage incontinence using kegel exercises follow the steps below:

i. First, ensure that your bladder is empty

ii. Sit on the floor and start to squeeze the kegel muscles

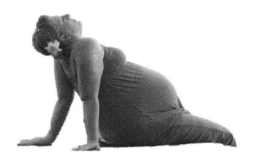

iii. Then, after about ten seconds, let the muscles relax for another ten seconds

iv. Repeat the process nine more times while sitting

v. Then, repeat ten times in a reclining position

vi. Stand up and repeat the process ten times

Note that the entire procedure should be done three times daily

# CHAPTER 5

## WHICH OTHER TIMES SHOULD YOU TRY KEGEL EXERCISES?

Aside from the problems mentioned so far, you can also perform kegel exercises during any of these periods:

*When you are pregnant:* Pregnant women can benefit a lot from performing kegels. Remember that pregnancy is one of the possible factors that cause loosening of the pelvic floor muscles.

**After childbirth**: Kegel exercises should also be done by women who have just recently delivered.

Childbearing can stretch the vaginal muscles, making them slightly lose their elasticity (even though it should regain its elastic nature naturally).

**_When menopause sets in_**: Menopause marks the end of menstruation in a woman. As a result, the pelvic floor muscles tend to lose their elasticity. This can be discomforting for women who still have an active sex life. To remedy the situation, such women should consider doing kegels.

***Before a hysterectomy***: A hysterectomy is a surgical operation to remove the uterus of a woman. Women who plan on doing this king of surgery can benefit from kegel exercises.

***After a hysterectomy***: Another good time to perform kegels is after a hysterectomy.

***When you have a prolapsed***: A prolapsed is when an internal or pelvic organ, like the uterus, falls out of its normal position. Pelvic organs can prolapse due to weakened pelvic floor muscles. Performing kegel exercises can help to correct the problem.

# CHAPTER 6

## WARNINGS AND PRECAUTIONS

You should not try to stop urinating every time you want to perform kegel exercises. This is because it can be counterproductive, and instead further weaken the pelvic muscles.

Ensure that your bladder is completely drained before you start the kegel exercises. This is necessary because you can leak urine while exercising, if your bladder is partially or completely full. Besides, doing kegel exercises on a filled bladder can cause you some pain.

Try not to overdo the exercises. That is you should try to be cautious while performing the kegel exercises and want to speed things up. This is because, like other forms of exercise, performing excess kegel exercises can injure the muscles.

In addition, women suffering from vaginismus are also advised not to perform kegel exercises. Vaginismus is a condition that is characterized by an involuntary contraction of the vagina.

It is also important that you keep other muscles in a relaxed position while squeezing your pelvic floor muscles. Common muscles that you may contract and that should be avoided are the buttock muscles and abdominal muscles.

If you have a health condition, it is also necessary that you discuss with your doctor before performing kegel exercises.

## People who should not try kegel exercises

Although kegel exercises offer great benefits to women, the exercises may not be effective in the following group of women:

Women with overflow incontinence. That is women who pass small quantities of urine unconsciously when they have a full bladder. When such women perform kegel exercises, instead of improving their condition, things get worse.

Also, we already mentioned that women with an underlying health condition should consult with a doctor before performing kegels. Hence, women in this category are advised not to try kegels, at least without a doctor's consent.

# REFERENCES

www.m.wikihow.com/Do-Kegel-Exercises

www.dailymail.co.uk/femail/article-4944356/The-five-exercises-that-make-vagina-tighter.html

www.mayoclinc.org/healty-lifestyle/womens-health/in-depth/kegel-exercises/art-20045283

www.health.havard.edu/bladder-and-bowel/step-by-step-guide-to-performing-kegel-exercises

www.healthline.com/health/kegel-exercises

www.punchng.com/three-steps-to-tightening-your-vagina-naturally

www.everydayhealth.com/incontinence/kegel-exercises-for-urinary-incontinence.aspx

www.pelvicexercises.com.au/pelvic-floor-exercises-1

www.mindbodygreen.com/0-26072/kegels-arent-enough-heres-what-you-should-be-doing-for-your-vagina.html

www.nhs.uk/common-health-questions/women-health/what-are-pelvic-floor-exercises/#pelvic-floor-exercises

www.cosmopolitan.com/sex-love/advice/g2285/kegel-exercises/

www.womenshealthmag.com/health/a18834773/how-to-do-kegels-right

www.womanlab.org/to-kegel-or-not-to-kegel-that-is-the-question

www.self.com/story/here-is-the-right-way-to-do-kegel-exercises

www.piplum.com/how-to/kegel-exercises-how-to-do-kegel-exercises-for-women-infographics

Printed in Great Britain
by Amazon

74303671R00029